Heart Health

Bible

by

Dr. Rachel Summers

Copyright no part of this book should be written copied or sold without Authors permission

Table Of Contents

Introduction: Understanding Cardiovascular Health 6
    Introduction to Cardiovascular Health 6
    Significance of a Healthy Heart 7
    Impact on Overall Well-being 8
    Statistics and Prevalence of Cardiovascular Conditions 9
    Global Burden of Cardiovascular Diseases 9
    Strokes and Their Impact 10
    Regional Variances and Demographic Trends 11
    National Burden 11
    Prevalence and Incidence 12
    Economic Impact 12
    Purpose of the Guide 13
    Objectives and Structure 13
    Emphasis on Holistic Wellness 15
    Empowering Lifestyle Changes 15

Chapter 1: Foundations of Cardiovascular Health 16
    Anatomy of the Heart 16
    Structure of the Heart 17
    Functions of the Heart 18
    Importance in Circulation 18
    Cardiovascular System Overview 19

Heart Health Bible

The Heart's Relationship with Blood Vessels 20
Blood Circulation and Its Significance 21
Interconnectedness and Coordination 22
Common Cardiovascular Conditions 22
Risk Factors Contributing to Cardiovascular Diseases . 27
1. Positive Effects (in moderate amounts): 41
2. Negative Effects (in excessive amounts): 41

Chapter 2: Dietary Plans for Heart Health 45
Principles of Heart-Healthy Eating 45
Sample 2 of a Mediterranean diet plan for a day: 58
DASH Diet: Dietary Approaches to Stop Hypertension 63
Nutritional Guidelines for Heart Health 71

1. Visual References: 72

2. Use Measuring Tools: 72

3. Read Labels: 73

4. Plate Division: 73

5. Mindful Eating: 73

6. Avoid Eating from Large Containers: 74

7. Plan and Prep Meals: 74

8. Practice Moderation: 74

9. Be Aware of Restaurant Portions: 74

Chapter 3: Exercise Routines for Cardiovascular Fitness 83
Importance of Physical Activity in Cardiovascular Health 83
Types of Exercises and Their Contributions to Heart Fitness 86

Chapter 4: Quitting Bad Habits 107
Step-by-step guide to help you quit smoking: 107
1. Recognize the Need for Change: 111

2. Set Realistic Goals: 111
3. Create a Plan: 112
4. Seek Support: 112
5. Find Alternative Coping Strategies: 112
6. Remove Temptations: 112
7. Stay Hydrated and Eat Healthily: 113
8. Educate Yourself: 113
9. Consider Professional Help: 113
10. Monitor Progress and Celebrate Milestones: 113

Chapter 5: Lifestyle Modifications for Heart Wellness. 118

Stress Management: Techniques for Reducing Stress and its Impact on Heart Health 118
1. Sleep Duration and Heart Health: 125
2. Influence on Heart Disease Risk: 126
3. Sleep and Inflammation: 126
4. Sleep Apnea and Heart Health: 127
5. Quality Sleep Tips for Heart Wellness: 127

Conclusion: 129

Let's recap the key points from each chapter: 129
Personalized Cardiovascular Wellness Plan 131
1. Dietary Modifications: 131
2. Physical Activity: 131
3. Stress Management: 132
4. Quality Sleep Improvement: 132
5. Risk Factor Management: 133
6. Regular Health Check-ups: 133
7. Accountability and Support: 134

Heart Health Bible

Introduction:

Understanding Cardiovascular Health

Introduction to Cardiovascular Health

A healthy heart stands as the cornerstone of vitality and well-being, serving as the engine that powers the body's intricate network of life-sustaining functions. Beyond its role as a muscular organ responsible for pumping blood throughout the body, the significance of a healthy heart transcends the boundaries of mere physicality, intertwining with our emotional, mental, and overall holistic wellness.

Significance of a Healthy Heart

The heart, tirelessly beating an average of 100,000 times a day, functions as the linchpin of our existence. Its optimal performance ensures the efficient circulation of oxygen and nutrients, vital for every cell, tissue, and organ. A robust and well-functioning cardiovascular system facilitates the transport of life-giving blood, regulating body temperature, supporting immune responses, and aiding in waste removal. A healthy heart is not merely a biological marvel; it embodies resilience, endurance, and the essence of life itself.

Impact on Overall Well-being

Beyond its physiological functions, the heart profoundly influences our overall well-being. A healthy heart is a harbinger of energy, enabling us to engage in daily activities with vigor and vitality. Conversely, cardiovascular ailments, if left unmanaged, can diminish our capacity to live life to its fullest. The impacts ripple through our lives, affecting physical capabilities, emotional equilibrium, mental clarity, and our ability to partake in the simplest pleasures life offers.

Statistics and Prevalence of Cardiovascular Conditions

Understanding the prevalence and impact of cardiovascular diseases is crucial in comprehending the magnitude of this global health challenge. Heart disease, strokes, and related cardiovascular conditions collectively stand as one of the leading causes of morbidity and mortality worldwide, affecting individuals across diverse demographics and geographic locations.

Global Burden of Cardiovascular Diseases

Statistics paint a stark reality: cardiovascular diseases account for a significant proportion of global health burdens. According to the World

Health Organization (WHO), heart disease claims the lives of over 17.9 million individuals annually, making it the leading cause of death globally. This figure encompasses various conditions such as coronary artery disease, heart attacks, heart failure, and arrhythmias, among others.

Strokes and Their Impact

In addition to heart diseases, strokes constitute a substantial portion of cardiovascular conditions. Each year, strokes cause around 6.2 million deaths worldwide, with millions more experiencing long-term disabilities due to stroke-related complications. These staggering numbers underscore the urgent need for preventative measures and effective management strategies to mitigate the impact of strokes on individuals and healthcare systems globally.

Regional Variances and Demographic Trends

The prevalence of cardiovascular diseases exhibits regional disparities and demographic variations. While these conditions affect individuals across all age groups and socio-economic backgrounds, certain regions and populations face a higher risk due to lifestyle factors, access to healthcare, genetic predispositions, and socio-economic determinants of health.

National Burden

In the United States, cardiovascular diseases remain a significant public health concern, exerting a substantial burden on both individuals and the healthcare system. The prevalence and impact of heart diseases, strokes, and related conditions contribute significantly to the nation's health challenges, affecting millions of Americans across diverse demographics.

Prevalence and Incidence

Heart disease stands as the leading cause of death in the United States. According to the Centers for Disease Control and Prevention (CDC), approximately 655,000 Americans die from heart disease each year, accounting for 1 in every 4 deaths. Moreover, an estimated 805,000 individuals experience heart attacks annually, underscoring the immediate and acute nature of this condition.

Economic Impact

The economic toll of cardiovascular diseases in the U.S. is staggering. The American Heart Association (AHA) estimates that heart disease and stroke account for an annual healthcare cost exceeding $200 billion. This financial burden encompasses direct medical expenses, lost productivity, and indirect costs associated with morbidity and disability caused by these conditions.

Purpose of the Guide

Welcome to the Healthy Hearts Manual: Comprehensive Guide to Cardiovascular Wellness. The purpose of this guide is to serve as a holistic resource, empowering individuals with the knowledge, tools, and strategies necessary to optimize their cardiovascular health and reduce the risks associated with heart diseases, strokes, and related conditions.

Objectives and Structure

This comprehensive guide is structured to provide a comprehensive understanding of cardiovascular health while emphasizing three fundamental pillars:

1. Dietary Plans: Exploring the impact of nutrition on heart health and presenting dietary guidelines, including the Mediterranean and DASH diets, tailored to support cardiovascular wellness.

2. Exercise Routines: Highlighting the significance of physical activity in maintaining heart health, offering diverse exercise routines suited for various fitness levels, and encouraging regular physical movement.

3. Risk Factor Management: Addressing modifiable risk factors such as hypertension, cholesterol levels, diabetes, smoking, stress, and their impact on cardiovascular well-being, accompanied by strategies for effective management.

Emphasis on Holistic Wellness

The core philosophy of this guide revolves around the belief that cardiovascular health extends beyond mere medical interventions. It encompasses a holistic approach that integrates lifestyle modifications, dietary choices, physical activity, and risk factor management to foster a healthier heart and, subsequently, a healthier life.

Empowering Lifestyle Changes

Our aim is to empower individuals to take charge of their cardiovascular health. By understanding the significance of dietary plans, adopting suitable exercise routines, and managing risk factors effectively, readers will be equipped with actionable insights to make informed choices, proactively enhance their heart health, and reduce the likelihood of cardiovascular diseases.

Chapter 1: Foundations of

Cardiovascular Health

Anatomy of the Heart

The human heart, a remarkable organ, serves as the epicenter of our circulatory system, orchestrating the continuous flow of life-giving blood throughout our bodies. Understanding the intricacies of its structure and functions unveils the awe-inspiring complexity behind this vital organ and underscores its paramount importance in sustaining our existence.

Structure of the Heart

The heart, nestled within the chest cavity and slightly tilted to the left, is roughly the size of a clenched fist. Comprising four chambers – two atria (upper chambers) and two ventricles (lower chambers) – the heart's design optimizes its ability to circulate blood effectively.

The atria serve as receiving chambers, accepting oxygen-depleted blood from the body into the right atrium and oxygen-rich blood from the lungs into the left atrium. Subsequently, the ventricles act as powerful pumps, propelling the blood out of the heart: the right ventricle sends deoxygenated blood to the lungs for oxygenation, while the left ventricle dispatches oxygenated blood to the entire body.

Functions of the Heart

The heart's primary function lies in its rhythmic contraction and relaxation, orchestrated by electrical impulses generated within its specialized tissues. This synchronized action, known as the cardiac cycle, propels blood through the circulatory system, ensuring a continuous supply of oxygen and nutrients to every cell, tissue, and organ in the body.

Importance in Circulation

The heart's role in circulation is pivotal. It works tirelessly, beating an average of 60 to 100 times per minute, approximately 100,000 times each day. Through its ceaseless efforts, the heart pumps nearly 5 to 6 liters of blood per minute, circulating the entire volume of blood through the body in less than a minute.

This systematic circulation ensures the delivery of vital oxygen and nutrients to tissues and organs, while simultaneously removing waste products such as carbon dioxide. The heart's intricate structure and meticulous coordination enable the body's survival, making it an indispensable hub in the symphony of life.

Cardiovascular System Overview

The cardiovascular system, an intricately woven network, encompasses the heart, blood vessels, and the vital fluid coursing through them. This remarkable system orchestrates the transportation of oxygen, nutrients, hormones, and cellular waste throughout the body, underscoring its paramount importance in sustaining life.

The Heart's Relationship with Blood Vessels

At the core of the cardiovascular system lies the heart, a powerhouse that propels blood through an extensive network of blood vessels. Arteries, veins, and capillaries form a vast infrastructure interconnecting the body's organs and tissues, facilitating the circulation of blood.

- Arteries: These vessels transport oxygenated blood away from the heart, delivering it to various parts of the body. They branch out into smaller vessels called arterioles, ensuring the distribution of nutrients and oxygen to tissues.

- Veins: Once the oxygen from the blood has been utilized by the body's tissues, the deoxygenated blood is carried back to the heart through veins. Veins progressively merge into larger vessels, eventually leading back to the heart.

- Capillaries: Microscopic vessels that form an intricate network between arteries and veins, facilitating the exchange of oxygen, nutrients, and waste products between blood and tissues.

Blood Circulation and Its Significance

Blood, the life-sustaining fluid, serves as the transport medium within the cardiovascular system. Its journey through the body is a continuous cycle – propelled by the heart's contractions, blood travels from the heart to the lungs for oxygenation, then back to the heart to be distributed to the entire body.

This cyclic movement ensures the nourishment and oxygenation of cells, tissues, and organs, while simultaneously removing waste products, maintaining the body's homeostasis, and supporting various physiological functions.

Interconnectedness and Coordination

The cardiovascular system operates as a unified entity, requiring seamless coordination between the heart, blood vessels, and blood itself. Each component plays a crucial role in maintaining the system's equilibrium, ensuring efficient circulation and sustaining the body's overall health.

Common Cardiovascular Conditions

Cardiovascular diseases encompass a spectrum of disorders affecting the heart and blood vessels, presenting multifaceted challenges to global health. These conditions, which range from heart diseases to strokes and related ailments, significantly impact individuals' health and well-being, warranting a comprehensive understanding and proactive preventive measures.

1. Coronary Artery Disease (CAD): CAD occurs due to the narrowing or blockage of the coronary arteries, usually caused by a buildup of plaque (atherosclerosis). Reduced blood flow to the heart muscles can result in chest pain (angina) or, in severe cases, a heart attack (myocardial infarction), where a portion of the heart muscle is damaged due to the lack of oxygenated blood.

2. Heart Failure: Heart failure happens when the heart becomes weak and cannot pump blood effectively. This may occur gradually over time due to conditions like CAD, hypertension, or heart valve disease. Symptoms include fatigue,

shortness of breath, swelling in the legs, and fluid retention.

3. Arrhythmias: Arrhythmias refer to irregular heartbeats that can cause the heart to beat too fast (tachycardia), too slow (bradycardia), or irregularly (atrial fibrillation). They may be harmless or life-threatening, leading to symptoms like palpitations, dizziness, fainting, or chest discomfort.

4. Stroke: Strokes occur when blood flow to the brain is disrupted, either due to a blockage in the blood vessels supplying the brain (ischemic stroke) or a rupture of blood vessels in the brain (hemorrhagic stroke). Symptoms include sudden numbness or weakness in the face, arm, or leg, confusion, trouble speaking or understanding speech, and severe headache.

5. Peripheral Artery Disease (PAD): PAD involves the narrowing of peripheral arteries, most commonly in the legs. Reduced blood flow can cause leg pain during physical activity

(claudication), sores that won't heal, and in severe cases, tissue damage or limb amputation.

6. Atherosclerosis: Atherosclerosis is the buildup of plaque (cholesterol, fat, calcium, and other substances) inside artery walls. This narrows the arteries and restricts blood flow, increasing the risk of heart attacks, strokes, and other cardiovascular problems.

7. Hypertension (High Blood Pressure): High blood pressure is a condition where the force of blood against artery walls is consistently too high. It can damage arteries, leading to heart disease, stroke, heart failure, kidney disease, and other health issues.

8. Cardiomyopathy: Cardiomyopathy refers to diseases of the heart muscle that weaken the heart's ability to pump blood. This condition can lead to heart enlargement, heart valve problems, and irregular heart rhythms.

9. Valvular Heart Disease: Valvular heart disease occurs when one or more heart valves fail to function properly, leading to stenosis (narrowing), regurgitation (leaking), or prolapse of the heart valves, affecting blood flow within the heart.

10. Congenital Heart Defects: These are structural heart abnormalities present at birth, such as holes in the heart, abnormal heart valves, or malformations of the heart's chambers or blood vessels. They can range from minor issues to severe, life-threatening conditions.

11. Pericardial Diseases: Conditions affecting the pericardium (the sac surrounding the heart) include pericarditis (inflammation of the pericardium) or pericardial effusion (accumulation of fluid in the pericardial sac), which can affect heart function.

12. Endocarditis: Endocarditis is an infection of the inner lining of the heart chambers and heart valves, usually caused by bacteria entering the

bloodstream. It can damage heart valves and impair heart function if left untreated.

Risk Factors Contributing to Cardiovascular Diseases

Cardiovascular diseases are influenced by an interplay of various factors, categorizable into modifiable and non-modifiable risk factors. Understanding these contributors is crucial in assessing one's susceptibility to heart-related ailments and formulating effective preventive strategies.

Non-Modifiable Risk Factors

1. Age: Age significantly impacts cardiovascular health due to the natural changes that occur in the heart and blood vessels over time. These age-related alterations contribute to an increased risk of cardiovascular diseases. Here's a detailed breakdown of how age affects cardiovascular health:

- Arterial Stiffness: With age, blood vessels gradually lose their elasticity and become stiffer. This reduced flexibility makes it harder for the vessels to expand and contract, leading to increased blood pressure. Arterial stiffness also affects the heart's workload, impacting its efficiency in pumping blood throughout the body.

- Atherosclerosis: Aging contributes to the development and progression of atherosclerosis, characterized by the accumulation of plaque in the artery walls.

Over time, plaque buildup narrows the arteries, restricting blood flow and increasing the risk of heart attacks and strokes.

- Heart Muscle Changes: The heart undergoes structural changes as one ages. It may slightly increase in size due to thickening of the walls of the heart's chambers. These changes can affect the heart's ability to pump blood efficiently and might contribute to conditions like heart failure or arrhythmias.

- Increased Risk Factors Over Time: As individuals age, they are more likely to accumulate other risk factors for cardiovascular diseases. For instance, they may have a longer exposure to unhealthy dietary patterns, sedentary lifestyles, smoking habits, or chronic stress, all of which can exacerbate the risk of heart-related issues.

- Reduced Heart Rate Variability: Aging is associated with a decrease in heart rate variability (HRV), the variation in the time intervals between heartbeats. Reduced HRV can be a marker of compromised heart health and an increased risk of cardiovascular events.

- Changes in Blood Vessel Function: Blood vessels lose some of their ability to dilate and constrict in response to various stimuli as individuals age. This impaired vascular function affects blood flow regulation and can contribute to hypertension and other cardiovascular problems.

- Risk of Other Health Conditions: As people age, they are more likely to develop other health conditions like diabetes, high blood pressure, or high cholesterol, all of which are significant risk factors for cardiovascular diseases.

2. Gender: Gender plays a significant role in cardiovascular health, influencing the risk, presentation, and outcomes of various heart-related conditions. Both men and women experience cardiovascular diseases, but the impact, symptoms, and risk factors may differ between the genders.

Gender Differences in Cardiovascular Health:

- Risk Profile: Traditionally, men have been considered at higher risk for cardiovascular diseases at a younger age compared to women. However, after menopause, a woman's risk of heart disease increases, and the risk gap narrows. Estrogen, which offers some protective effects on heart health, declines after menopause, contributing to increased risk.

- Symptom Presentation: Women may experience different symptoms of heart disease than men. While chest pain (angina) is a common symptom in both genders, women might also present with atypical symptoms such as shortness of breath, nausea, vomiting, back or jaw pain, and extreme fatigue. This variation in symptom presentation can lead to underdiagnosis and delayed treatment in women.

- Types of Heart Disease: Some heart conditions may affect men and women differently. For instance, women may have a higher risk of developing microvascular disease, which affects the small arteries in the heart. Additionally, women are more prone to certain types of heart conditions like Takotsubo cardiomyopathy (also known as broken heart syndrome), which can be triggered by extreme emotional or physical stress.

- Risk Factors: The distribution and impact of risk factors can differ between genders. For example, diabetes tends to have a more detrimental effect on heart health in women compared to men. Women with diabetes have a higher risk of heart disease than diabetic men. Additionally, hormonal factors, including pregnancy complications like gestational diabetes or preeclampsia, can also impact a woman's future cardiovascular health.

- Diagnostic Challenges: Historically, heart disease has been more extensively studied in men, leading to potential diagnostic challenges in women. Diagnostic tests and treatment protocols may be based on studies primarily involving male subjects, potentially affecting the accuracy of diagnosis and treatment strategies for women.

3. Family History: Family history of cardiovascular diseases plays a crucial role in assessing an

individual's susceptibility to heart-related ailments. Understanding this aspect involves examining the influence of genetic predispositions and shared environmental factors among family members.

- Genetic Predisposition: Genetics can significantly impact an individual's risk of developing cardiovascular diseases. If close blood relatives, such as parents or siblings, have a history of heart disease, heart attacks, strokes, or related conditions, there's an increased likelihood that other family members may also be predisposed to these ailments. This genetic predisposition doesn't guarantee the development of cardiovascular disease but raises the risk.

- Inherited Traits: Certain inherited traits or genetic mutations can influence cholesterol metabolism, blood pressure regulation, clotting mechanisms, and heart muscle structure, among other factors. For instance, familial hypercholesterolemia, an inherited condition causing high levels of LDL cholesterol, can lead to premature heart disease if left untreated.

- Shared Environmental Factors: Apart from genetics, shared environmental factors within families can also contribute to increased heart disease risk. Families often share lifestyle habits, dietary patterns, exercise routines, and exposure to stress or environmental toxins, which collectively influence cardiovascular health.

Modifiable Risk Factors

1. Tobacco Use: Tobacco use significantly impacts cardiovascular health through a complex pathophysiological process that affects various systems within the body. The constituents of tobacco smoke, including nicotine, tar, carbon monoxide, and numerous other harmful

chemicals, exert detrimental effects on the cardiovascular system.

Pathophysiological Effects of Tobacco Use on Cardiovascular Health:

- Damage to Blood Vessels: The chemicals in tobacco smoke damage the inner lining of blood vessels, initiating an inflammatory response. This leads to the formation of plaque (atherosclerosis) inside the arteries, causing them to narrow and harden over time. Atherosclerosis reduces blood flow to the heart, brain, and other vital organs.

- Increased Risk of Clot Formation: Tobacco smoke can trigger the formation of blood clots (thrombosis) by promoting platelet aggregation and altering the balance of clotting factors in the blood. Clots can obstruct blood vessels, leading to heart attacks or strokes.

- Elevated Blood Pressure: Nicotine, a primary component of tobacco, raises blood pressure by constricting blood vessels and increasing heart rate. Elevated blood pressure strains the heart and blood vessels, increasing the risk of heart diseases and strokes.

- Damaging Effects on Cholesterol Levels: Smoking can lower HDL ("good") cholesterol levels while simultaneously raising LDL ("bad") cholesterol levels. This imbalance contributes to the buildup of plaque in arteries, fostering atherosclerosis.

- Reduced Oxygen Delivery: Carbon monoxide, present in tobacco smoke, binds more readily to hemoglobin than oxygen, reducing the blood's capacity to carry oxygen. This results in decreased oxygen delivery to the body's tissues and organs, including the heart, compromising their function.

- Impact on Heart Rhythm: Tobacco use can disrupt the normal rhythm of the heart, leading to arrhythmias such as atrial fibrillation, which can increase the risk of blood clots and stroke.

- Endothelial Dysfunction: Tobacco smoke damages the endothelial cells lining blood vessels, compromising their ability to regulate blood flow, vascular tone, and inflammation. This dysfunction contributes to the progression of atherosclerosis.

- Overall Inflammatory Response: Tobacco smoke triggers a systemic inflammatory response within the body, promoting the release of inflammatory cytokines and other substances that further damage blood vessels and contribute to cardiovascular diseases.

2. Unhealthy Diet: Diets high in saturated fats, trans fats, cholesterol, sodium, and added sugars contribute to obesity, high blood pressure, and high cholesterol, increasing the risk of heart diseases.

3. Physical Inactivity: Lack of regular physical activity is associated with various cardiovascular conditions. Exercise helps maintain a healthy weight, lowers blood pressure, and improves heart health.

4. Obesity and Body Composition: Being overweight or obese increases the risk of developing cardiovascular diseases. Excess weight strains the heart, raises blood pressure, and affects cholesterol levels.

5. High Blood Pressure: Hypertension is a significant risk factor for heart disease and stroke. It strains the heart and damages blood vessels over time, leading to various cardiovascular complications.

6. High Cholesterol Levels: Elevated levels of LDL ("bad") cholesterol and low levels of HDL ("good") cholesterol increase the risk of atherosclerosis and heart diseases.

7. Diabetes: Individuals with diabetes have a higher risk of developing cardiovascular diseases due to factors like high blood sugar levels damaging blood vessels and nerves.

8. Stress: Chronic stress can contribute to heart disease risk through various mechanisms, including increased blood pressure, unhealthy coping mechanisms (like smoking or overeating), and inflammation.

9. Alcohol Consumption: Alcohol consumption, while often associated with social gatherings or relaxation, can impact cardiovascular health in various ways. The pathophysiological effects of alcohol on the cardiovascular system involve both positive and negative aspects, depending on the amount consumed and individual factors.

Effects of Alcohol on Cardiovascular Health:

1. Positive Effects (in moderate amounts):

- *Increase in HDL Cholesterol: Moderate alcohol intake has been linked to higher levels of high-density lipoprotein (HDL) cholesterol, often referred to as "good" cholesterol. HDL cholesterol helps remove excess cholesterol from the blood, reducing the risk of atherosclerosis.*

- *Antioxidant Properties: Certain alcoholic beverages, such as red wine, contain antioxidants like resveratrol, which may have protective effects on the heart by reducing inflammation and preventing blood clot formation.*

2. Negative Effects (in excessive amounts):

- Hypertension (High Blood Pressure): Chronic heavy alcohol consumption can lead to hypertension. Alcohol affects the sympathetic nervous system, causing increased heart rate and vasoconstriction, which raises blood pressure over time.

- Cardiomyopathy: Prolonged excessive alcohol consumption can weaken the heart muscles, leading to cardiomyopathy (alcoholic cardiomyopathy). This condition results in the heart's reduced ability to pump blood effectively, potentially leading to heart failure.

- Arrhythmias: Alcohol abuse can cause irregular heart rhythms (arrhythmias), including atrial fibrillation, which increases the risk of stroke and other cardiovascular complications.

- Atherosclerosis: Heavy drinking can contribute to the development of atherosclerosis, the buildup of plaque in arteries, by increasing levels of triglycerides and promoting inflammation, which can lead to narrowed or blocked arteries.

- Heart Failure: Excessive alcohol consumption can directly damage the heart muscle, leading to dilated cardiomyopathy and eventual heart failure.

Pathophysiological Mechanisms:

- Impact on Heart Muscle: Chronic alcohol consumption can cause direct toxicity to heart muscle cells, impairing their function and structure. This may lead to weakened contractions, enlarged heart chambers, and reduced pumping ability.

- Effect on Blood Pressure: Alcohol can disrupt the balance of the sympathetic and parasympathetic nervous systems, leading to increased sympathetic activity. This results in vasoconstriction and increased heart rate, contributing to elevated blood pressure.

- Disruption of Lipid Profiles: Heavy drinking can alter lipid metabolism, leading to increased triglycerides and reduced HDL cholesterol, promoting atherosclerosis and plaque formation in arteries.

- Electrolyte Imbalance: Alcohol can disrupt electrolyte balance in the body, leading to changes in sodium and potassium levels, which may affect heart rhythm and function.

Chapter 2: Dietary Plans for Heart Health

Principles of Heart-Healthy Eating

A heart-healthy diet is a cornerstone in the prevention and management of cardiovascular diseases. It focuses on fostering overall health by making informed dietary choices that prioritize heart health and general well-being. Emphasizing balanced nutrition and mindful eating habits forms the bedrock of a heart-healthy diet.

Key Elements of a Heart-Healthy Diet:

1. Fruits and Vegetables: Incorporating a variety of colorful fruits and vegetables provides essential vitamins, minerals, fiber, and antioxidants. These nutrients help reduce inflammation, lower blood pressure, and improve overall cardiovascular health.

2. Whole Grains: Opting for whole grains such as brown rice, whole wheat bread, oats, quinoa, and barley over refined grains helps maintain healthy cholesterol levels, stabilizes blood sugar, and provides sustained energy due to their fiber content.

3. Healthy Fats: Including sources of healthy fats like avocados, nuts, seeds, olive oil, and fatty fish (e.g., salmon, mackerel, and trout) rich in omega-3 fatty acids supports heart health by reducing inflammation and lowering cholesterol levels.

4. Lean Proteins: Choosing lean protein sources, including poultry, fish, legumes, tofu, and low-fat dairy products, instead of fatty meats, helps maintain a healthy weight and supports heart health.

5. Limiting Saturated and Trans Fats: Reducing the intake of saturated fats found in processed foods, red meat, and full-fat dairy products, as well as eliminating trans fats often present in fried foods and commercially baked goods, is crucial in preventing plaque buildup in arteries.

6. Reducing Sodium Intake: Lowering sodium consumption by minimizing processed and packaged foods and opting for fresh, whole foods helps manage blood pressure and reduces the risk of heart diseases.

7. Moderation with Sugar and Added Sweeteners: Limiting added sugars and sweetened beverages is essential for overall health. Excessive sugar

intake contributes to weight gain, inflammation, and increased risk of heart diseases.

Mindful Eating Habits:

1. Portion Control: Being mindful of portion sizes helps prevent overeating and supports weight management, a crucial aspect of heart health.

2. Eating Patterns: Adopting a balanced eating pattern, such as the Mediterranean or DASH (Dietary Approaches to Stop Hypertension) diet, emphasizes whole foods, fruits, vegetables, and lean proteins, promoting heart health.

3. Hydration: Staying adequately hydrated by consuming water and limiting sugary drinks contributes to overall well-being and supports heart health.

Mediterranean Diet: The Heart's Ally

The Mediterranean diet, renowned for its potential in promoting heart health and overall well-being, draws inspiration from the dietary patterns of countries bordering the Mediterranean Sea. This diet isn't merely a regimen but a way of life, encompassing a diverse array of foods and lifestyle practices that have garnered attention for their positive impact on cardiovascular wellness.

Key Components of the Mediterranean Diet:

1. Abundance of Plant-Based Foods: The Mediterranean diet centers around whole, plant-based foods such as fruits, vegetables, legumes,

nuts, seeds, and whole grains. These nutrient-dense foods provide essential vitamins, minerals, fiber, and antioxidants, contributing to reduced inflammation and improved heart health.

2. Healthy Fats: Emphasis is placed on consuming healthy fats, particularly monounsaturated fats found in olive oil, avocados, and nuts, as well as omega-3 fatty acids sourced from fatty fish like salmon and mackerel. These fats support cardiovascular health by reducing cholesterol levels and inflammation.

3. Moderate Consumption of Dairy and Poultry: The Mediterranean diet encourages moderate consumption of dairy products, focusing on low-fat or fat-free options, and poultry as sources of lean protein, limiting red meat intake.

4. Regular Intake of Fish: Fish, especially oily varieties like salmon, sardines, and mackerel rich in omega-3 fatty acids, is a staple in the Mediterranean diet. Regular fish consumption

supports heart health and reduces the risk of cardiovascular diseases.

5. Minimal Red Meat and Processed Foods: Reducing the intake of red meat and processed foods, which are high in saturated fats and sodium, is a fundamental aspect of this diet. This practice helps lower cholesterol levels and maintains blood pressure within a healthy range.

6. Herbs, Spices, and Flavorful Additions: Herbs and spices like basil, oregano, garlic, and cinnamon are used liberally in Mediterranean cuisine, enhancing flavor without relying on excessive salt or unhealthy condiments.

Benefits of the Mediterranean Diet in Cardiovascular Wellness:

1. Heart Disease Prevention: Numerous studies have shown that adhering to the Mediterranean

diet can reduce the risk of heart disease, stroke, and heart attacks due to its focus on heart-healthy foods.

2. Improved Lipid Profile: This dietary pattern has been associated with increased HDL cholesterol (the "good" cholesterol) and decreased LDL cholesterol (the "bad" cholesterol), promoting better lipid profiles and reduced plaque buildup in arteries.

3. Blood Pressure Management: The Mediterranean diet's emphasis on whole foods, healthy fats, and lower sodium intake has shown positive effects on managing blood pressure levels, contributing to better heart health.

4. Reduced Inflammation: The abundance of antioxidants and anti-inflammatory compounds in the Mediterranean diet aids in reducing inflammation, a key contributor to various cardiovascular conditions.

Sample 1 of a Mediterranean diet plan for a day:

Breakfast:

- Greek Yogurt Parfait:
  - Ingredients:
    - 1 cup Greek yogurt (low-fat or non-fat)
    - 1/2 cup mixed berries (blueberries, strawberries, raspberries)
    - 1 tablespoon honey or a sprinkle of chopped nuts (optional)
  - Instructions:
    - In a bowl or glass, layer Greek yogurt with mixed berries.
    - Drizzle honey or sprinkle nuts on top for added flavor (optional).

- Whole Grain Toast with Avocado:
  - Ingredients:
    - 2 slices whole grain bread

- 1 ripe avocado
   - Pinch of sea salt and black pepper
  - Instructions:
   - Toast the whole grain bread.
   - Mash the ripe avocado and spread it over the toast.
   - Sprinkle with a pinch of sea salt and black pepper for taste.

Mid-Morning Snack:

- Mixed Nuts and Fresh Fruit:
  - Ingredients:
   - 1 handful of mixed nuts (almonds, walnuts, pistachios)
   - 1 apple or an orange
  - Instructions:
   - Enjoy a handful of mixed nuts with a fresh apple or orange.

Lunch:

- Mediterranean Chickpea Salad:
  - Ingredients:
    - 1 can chickpeas (rinsed and drained)
    - 1 cucumber (diced)
    - 1 bell pepper (diced)
    - 1/2 red onion (finely chopped)
    - Cherry tomatoes (halved)
    - Kalamata olives (pitted)
    - Feta cheese (optional)
    - Fresh parsley (chopped)
    - Dressing: Olive oil, lemon juice, garlic, salt, and pepper
  - Instructions:
    - In a large bowl, combine chickpeas, cucumber, bell pepper, onion, cherry tomatoes, and olives.
    - Crumble feta cheese (optional) over the salad.
    - In a separate bowl, whisk together olive oil, lemon juice, minced garlic, salt, and pepper to create the dressing.

- Toss the salad with the dressing and garnish with fresh parsley.

Afternoon Snack:

- Whole Grain Crackers with Hummus:
  - Ingredients:
    - Whole grain crackers
    - Hummus (store-bought or homemade)
  - Instructions:
    - Enjoy a serving of whole grain crackers with a side of hummus.

Dinner:

- Grilled Salmon with Roasted Vegetables:
  - Ingredients:
    - Salmon fillet (fresh or thawed)
    - Assorted vegetables (bell peppers, zucchini, eggplant, cherry tomatoes)
    - Olive oil, garlic, dried herbs (rosemary, thyme)

- Lemon wedges
 - Instructions:
   - Preheat the grill or oven.
   - Season the salmon fillet with olive oil, garlic, herbs, salt, and pepper.
   - Grill or bake the salmon until cooked through.
   - Toss the assorted vegetables with olive oil, salt, and pepper. Roast them until tender.
   - Serve the grilled salmon with roasted vegetables and a squeeze of fresh lemon.

Evening Snack (Optional):

- Fresh Fruit Salad:
  - Ingredients:
    - Assorted fresh fruits (strawberries, kiwi, pineapple, grapes)
    - Mint leaves (optional)
  - Instructions:
    - Chop the fresh fruits into bite-sized pieces and combine them in a bowl.

- Garnish with mint leaves for added freshness (optional).

Sample 2 of a Mediterranean diet plan for a day:

Breakfast:

- Mediterranean Omelette:
  - Ingredients:
    - 2 eggs
    - Spinach leaves
    - Diced tomatoes
    - Feta cheese (optional)
    - Chopped fresh basil
    - Olive oil
  - Instructions:
    - In a bowl, whisk the eggs.
    - Heat olive oil in a pan, add spinach and diced tomatoes, and sauté for a few minutes.
    - Pour the whisked eggs over the vegetables and cook until the omelette sets.
    - Sprinkle crumbled feta cheese and chopped basil on top before folding the omelette.

- Whole Grain Toast with Olive Tapenade:
  - Ingredients:
    - 2 slices whole grain bread
    - Olive tapenade (store-bought or homemade)
  - Instructions:
    - Toast the whole grain bread.
    - Spread olive tapenade over the toast for a flavorful topping.

Mid-Morning Snack:

- Greek Yogurt with Honey and Almonds:
  - Ingredients:
    - Greek yogurt (low-fat or non-fat)
    - Drizzle of honey
    - Sliced almonds
  - Instructions:
    - Serve Greek yogurt in a bowl.
    - Drizzle honey over the yogurt and sprinkle sliced almonds for added crunch.

Lunch:

- Mediterranean Quinoa Salad:
  - Ingredients:
    - Cooked quinoa
    - Diced cucumber
    - Cherry tomatoes (halved)
    - Chopped red onion
    - Diced bell pepper (any color)
    - Kalamata olives (pitted and sliced)
    - Fresh parsley (chopped)
    - Feta cheese
    - Dressing: Olive oil, lemon juice, minced garlic, salt, and pepper
  - Instructions:
    - In a large bowl, combine cooked quinoa, cucumber, tomatoes, onion, bell pepper, olives, and parsley.
    - Crumble feta cheese over the salad.
    - Whisk together olive oil, lemon juice, minced garlic, salt, and pepper to make the dressing. Toss the salad with the dressing.

Afternoon Snack:

- Hummus with Sliced Vegetables:
  - Ingredients:
    - Hummus (store-bought or homemade)
    - Sliced bell peppers, carrots, and cucumber
  - Instructions:
    - Enjoy hummus with sliced vegetables as a healthy and flavorful snack.

Dinner:

- Mediterranean Baked Chicken with Roasted Vegetables:
  - Ingredients:
    - Chicken breasts or thighs
    - Cherry tomatoes
    - Red onion (cut into wedges)
    - Bell peppers (sliced)
    - Kalamata olives

- Olive oil, garlic, dried oregano, salt, and pepper
  - Instructions:
    - Preheat the oven and prepare a baking dish.
    - Season the chicken with olive oil, garlic, oregano, salt, and pepper.
    - Place the seasoned chicken in the baking dish surrounded by cherry tomatoes, onion, bell peppers, and olives.
    - Bake until the chicken is cooked through and the vegetables are tender.

Evening Snack (Optional):

- Mixed Berries with Greek Yogurt:
  - Ingredients:
    - Mixed berries (blueberries, strawberries, raspberries)
    - Greek yogurt (low-fat or non-fat)
  - Instructions:
    - Serve a bowl of mixed berries with a side of Greek yogurt for a refreshing snack.

DASH Diet: Dietary Approaches to Stop Hypertension

The Dietary Approaches to Stop Hypertension (DASH) diet is a dietary pattern specifically designed to reduce high blood pressure (hypertension) and promote heart health. It emphasizes a balanced and nutritious eating plan focused on whole foods, aiming to lower blood pressure and reduce the risk of cardiovascular diseases.

Key Components of the DASH Diet:

1. Rich in Fruits and Vegetables: The DASH diet emphasizes a high intake of fruits and vegetables, which are rich in vitamins, minerals, fiber, and antioxidants. These nutrients contribute to

reducing blood pressure and improving overall heart health.

2. Whole Grains: Whole grains such as brown rice, whole wheat bread, oats, barley, and quinoa form an essential part of the DASH diet. They provide complex carbohydrates, fiber, and various nutrients beneficial for heart health.

3. Lean Protein Sources: The diet recommends including lean sources of protein, such as poultry, fish, beans, legumes, and nuts. These protein sources are lower in saturated fats and support heart health.

4. Low-Fat Dairy Products: The DASH diet encourages the consumption of low-fat or fat-free dairy products like milk, yogurt, and cheese. These dairy products are excellent sources of calcium, potassium, and protein without the added saturated fats.

5. Limited Saturated Fats and Added Sugars: Reducing the intake of foods high in saturated

fats, such as fatty meats and full-fat dairy products, as well as limiting added sugars and sugary beverages, is a fundamental aspect of the DASH diet.

6. Moderate Sodium Intake: The DASH diet recommends limiting sodium intake to help control blood pressure. Reducing the consumption of processed and packaged foods high in sodium is emphasized.

Impact of the DASH Diet on Heart Health:

1. Blood Pressure Management: The DASH diet has shown effectiveness in lowering blood pressure, particularly in individuals with hypertension. The emphasis on whole foods, potassium-rich fruits and vegetables, and reduced sodium intake contributes to blood pressure control.

2. Improved Lipid Profile: Adherence to the DASH diet has been associated with favorable changes in lipid profiles, including lower levels of LDL cholesterol and higher levels of HDL cholesterol, supporting heart health.

3. Reduced Cardiovascular Risk: Studies have indicated that following the DASH diet can reduce the risk of developing cardiovascular diseases, including heart attacks and strokes, by promoting a heart-healthy eating pattern.

Sample of a one-day meal plan based on the principles of the DASH diet:

Breakfast:

- Vegetable Omelette:
  - Ingredients:
    - 2 eggs
    - Chopped spinach, tomatoes, bell peppers
    - Onion (diced)
    - Low-fat cheese (optional)
    - Olive oil
  - Instructions:
    - Sauté chopped vegetables in olive oil until tender.
    - Beat eggs and pour them over the cooked vegetables in a pan.
    - Sprinkle low-fat cheese if desired.

- Cook until the omelette is set and fold it over.

- Whole Grain Toast:
  - Serve with a slice of whole grain toast.

- Fresh Fruit Salad:
  - Assorted fresh fruits like berries, oranges, and melons.

Mid-Morning Snack:

- Greek Yogurt with Berries:
  - Plain Greek yogurt topped with mixed berries.

Lunch:

- Grilled Chicken Salad:
  - Grilled chicken breast (skinless)
  - Mixed greens (spinach, lettuce)
  - Cucumber, cherry tomatoes, bell peppers
  - Olive oil and balsamic vinegar as dressing

- Whole Wheat Pita Bread:
  - Serve with a whole wheat pita bread on the side.

Afternoon Snack:

- Mixed Nuts:
  - A handful of unsalted mixed nuts (almonds, walnuts, pistachios).

Dinner:

- Baked Salmon with Vegetables:
  - Baked salmon fillet seasoned with herbs, lemon juice, and olive oil.
  - Steamed or roasted mixed vegetables (such as broccoli, carrots, and asparagus).

- Brown Rice:
  - Serve with a side of cooked brown rice.

Evening Snack (Optional):

- Apple Slices with Almond Butter:
  - Sliced apple with a tablespoon of almond butter.

Fluids throughout the day:

- Water: Aim to drink at least 8 cups (64 ounces) of water or more per day.
- Herbal Teas: Enjoy herbal teas without added sugar for variety and hydration.

Nutritional Guidelines for Heart Health

Optimal heart health is not solely about what foods to include in the diet but also about understanding essential nutritional guidelines that contribute to overall well-being. Adopting healthy eating habits and adhering to specific dietary recommendations can significantly impact cardiovascular health.

Portion Control:

Portion control is a fundamental aspect of maintaining a balanced diet and supporting overall health, including heart health. It involves being mindful of the amount of food consumed at meals and snacks. Understanding portion sizes helps prevent overeating, promotes weight management, and ensures a well-balanced intake of nutrients.

Here are some detailed tips on portion control:

1. Visual References:
   - Use visual cues to estimate portion sizes. For instance:
      - A serving of protein (meat, fish, poultry) should be about the size of your palm or a deck of cards.
      - A serving of grains or starchy foods like rice or pasta should match the size of a tennis ball.
      - A serving of fats (like butter or oil) should be about the size of your thumb.

2. Use Measuring Tools:
   - Initially, use measuring cups, spoons, or a food scale to accurately measure serving sizes.

This helps familiarize you with appropriate portion sizes for different foods.

3. Read Labels:
   - Pay attention to serving sizes listed on food labels. Sometimes the packaging may contain multiple servings, and consuming the entire package can result in overeating.

4. Plate Division:
   - Divide your plate visually to ensure a balanced meal:
     - Allocate half the plate for vegetables and fruits.
     - One-quarter of the plate for lean protein sources.
     - One-quarter for whole grains or starchy foods.

5. Mindful Eating:
   - Eat slowly, and pay attention to hunger and fullness cues. Pause between bites, chew thoroughly, and savor the flavors. This allows

your body to recognize when it's full, preventing overeating.

6. Avoid Eating from Large Containers:
   - Instead of eating directly from large packages or containers, portion out a serving size into a bowl or plate. This prevents mindless eating and helps control portions.

7. Plan and Prep Meals:
   - Preparing meals in advance or using meal prep containers can assist in portion control by ensuring you have predetermined, appropriately sized portions ready to eat.

8. Practice Moderation:
   - It's not about deprivation but moderation. Enjoying occasional treats in smaller portions can help satisfy cravings without overindulging.

9. Be Aware of Restaurant Portions:
   - Restaurant portions tend to be larger than recommended serving sizes. Consider sharing meals, ordering appetizers as a main dish, or

packing half the meal to-go to control portion sizes.

By incorporating these strategies into your daily eating habits, you can effectively manage portion sizes, improve awareness of food intake, and maintain a balanced diet conducive to better heart health and overall well-being.

Reducing Sodium Intake:

Reducing sodium intake is a crucial aspect of a heart-healthy diet due to its direct correlation with elevated blood pressure and increased risk of cardiovascular diseases. Here's a detailed explanation of how to effectively reduce sodium intake:

Understanding Sodium and Its Effects:

Sodium is an essential mineral required by the body for various functions, including maintaining fluid balance, transmitting nerve impulses, and aiding muscle contractions. However, excessive sodium consumption, primarily in the form of sodium chloride (table salt), can lead to health issues, particularly concerning heart health.

Effects of High Sodium Intake on Heart Health:

- Increased Blood Pressure: Excessive sodium intake can cause the body to retain more water, leading to increased blood volume and subsequently higher blood pressure. Elevated blood pressure strains the heart and blood vessels, increasing the risk of heart diseases, strokes, and kidney problems.

Steps to Reduce Sodium Intake:

1. Read Food Labels: Be mindful of packaged and processed foods as they often contain high levels of sodium. Check nutrition labels and opt for products with lower sodium content. Aim for items labeled as "low-sodium," "reduced sodium," or "no added salt."

2. Choose Fresh Foods: Incorporate more fresh, whole foods into your diet. Fruits, vegetables, lean meats, fish, and poultry naturally contain lower levels of sodium compared to processed alternatives.

3. Limit Processed Foods: Highly processed foods such as canned soups, processed meats (like bacon, sausages, and deli meats), instant noodles, sauces, and condiments tend to have higher

sodium content. Limiting their intake can significantly reduce overall sodium consumption.

4. Use Herbs and Spices: Flavor your meals with herbs, spices, citrus, and other seasonings instead of relying solely on salt. Experiment with flavorful combinations to enhance taste without adding excess sodium.

5. Cook at Home: Prepare meals at home whenever possible. This way, you have better control over the ingredients and can reduce salt while cooking. Limit the use of salt during cooking and offer it sparingly at the table.

6. Be Cautious Eating Out: When dining out, ask for dishes with less salt or sauces on the side. Restaurants often use high amounts of salt in their recipes for flavor, so it's essential to be mindful of this when dining out.

7. Gradual Reduction: Gradually reduce your sodium intake rather than making sudden drastic

changes. Your taste buds will gradually adjust to less salty flavors over time.

Recommended Sodium Intake:

The American Heart Association recommends consuming no more than 2,300 milligrams (mg) of sodium per day, with an ideal limit of 1,500 mg per day for most adults, especially those with high blood pressure or at risk for heart diseases. However, most individuals consume well over these recommended levels due to the prevalence of processed foods in modern diets.

Conclusion:

By being aware of sources of dietary sodium and making conscious choices to limit its intake, individuals can take proactive steps toward reducing their risk of cardiovascular diseases, maintaining healthy blood pressure levels, and overall promoting better heart health.

Incorporating Heart-Friendly Nutrients:

Certain nutrients play a pivotal role in supporting heart health. Including these nutrients in the diet can have beneficial effects:

1. Omega-3 Fatty Acids: Found in fatty fish (such as salmon, mackerel, and sardines), flaxseeds, chia seeds, and walnuts, omega-3 fatty acids contribute to reducing inflammation and improving heart health.

2. Potassium: Foods rich in potassium, like bananas, oranges, spinach, potatoes, and yogurt, can help regulate blood pressure and counteract the effects of sodium in the body.

3. Magnesium: Magnesium-rich foods such as nuts, seeds, whole grains, leafy greens, and legumes support heart health by assisting in muscle function and regulating blood pressure.

4. Fiber: Incorporating fiber-rich foods like whole grains, fruits, vegetables, legumes, and nuts aids in lowering cholesterol levels and maintaining a healthy weight, benefiting heart health.

5. Antioxidants: Antioxidants, present in colorful fruits and vegetables, help combat oxidative stress and reduce inflammation, promoting heart health.

Balanced Nutrition for Heart Health:

Embracing a balanced and varied diet that encompasses these nutritional guidelines, while emphasizing whole, unprocessed foods, lean proteins, healthy fats, and a rainbow of fruits and vegetables, lays the foundation for a heart-healthy lifestyle. Coupled with portion control and mindful eating, these guidelines can significantly contribute to maintaining optimal cardiovascular wellness.

Chapter 3: Exercise Routines for Cardiovascular Fitness

Importance of Physical Activity in Cardiovascular Health

Physical activity plays a pivotal role in maintaining optimal cardiovascular health and reducing the risks associated with heart diseases. Its significance extends beyond enhancing physical fitness; regular exercise positively impacts various aspects of overall well-being, specifically targeting heart health.

Key Roles of Exercise in Cardiovascular Health:

1. Strengthening the Heart Muscle: Engaging in regular physical activity, particularly aerobic exercises like brisk walking, jogging, cycling, or swimming, challenges the heart to pump blood more efficiently, thereby strengthening the heart muscle.

2. Improving Circulation: Exercise promotes better circulation by enhancing the body's ability to transport oxygen-rich blood to the muscles and vital organs. This improved blood flow supports the heart and reduces strain on the cardiovascular system.

3. Lowering Blood Pressure: Regular physical activity contributes to reducing high blood pressure, a significant risk factor for heart diseases. It helps maintain healthy blood pressure

levels by increasing the flexibility of blood vessels and reducing their resistance.

4. Managing Cholesterol Levels: Exercise plays a role in improving the lipid profile by increasing high-density lipoprotein (HDL or "good" cholesterol) and lowering low-density lipoprotein (LDL or "bad" cholesterol), thereby reducing the risk of plaque buildup in the arteries.

5. Controlling Weight: Physical activity aids in weight management and prevents obesity, which is associated with an increased risk of heart diseases. Exercise helps burn calories, build lean muscle mass, and maintain a healthy body weight.

6. Reducing Stress and Improving Mental Health: Regular exercise has positive effects on mental health by reducing stress, anxiety, and depression. A healthy mind contributes to overall well-being, indirectly benefiting heart health.

7. Enhancing Overall Cardiovascular Fitness: Consistent engagement in exercise routines improves endurance, stamina, and overall cardiovascular fitness, enabling the heart to function optimally.

Types of Exercises and Their Contributions to Heart Fitness

1. Aerobic Exercises:

Definition: Aerobic exercises, also known as cardiovascular or cardio exercises, involve rhythmic and continuous movements that elevate the heart rate and increase oxygen consumption. These activities primarily target the cardiovascular system, enhancing heart and lung function.

Contributions to Heart Fitness:

- Improved Heart Health: Aerobic exercises challenge the heart by making it work harder to pump oxygenated blood throughout the body. Over time, this strengthens the heart muscle and improves its efficiency.

- Enhanced Endurance: Regular participation in aerobic activities boosts endurance levels, allowing the body to perform physical tasks for longer periods without fatigue. This endurance is directly related to heart fitness and improved cardiovascular function.

- Lowered Blood Pressure: Engaging in aerobic exercises helps regulate blood pressure by promoting better blood vessel flexibility and reducing stress on the heart.

- Better Cholesterol Levels: Aerobic activities aid in raising HDL ("good") cholesterol levels while reducing LDL ("bad") cholesterol levels, contributing to better heart health.

- Examples: Running, brisk walking, cycling, swimming, dancing, rowing, and aerobic classes are common aerobic exercises that significantly benefit heart fitness.

Step-by-step procedure for common aerobic exercises:

Brisk Walking:

1. Warm-up: Start with a 5-10 minute warm-up by walking at a comfortable pace to prepare your muscles for the exercise.
2. Increase Pace: Gradually increase your walking pace to a brisk speed. Swing your arms naturally as you walk.
3. Maintain Posture: Keep an upright posture, looking forward, not down at your feet. Engage

your core muscles and keep your shoulders relaxed.

4. Breathe: Breathe deeply and rhythmically as you walk, inhaling through your nose and exhaling through your mouth.

5. Duration: Aim for at least 30 minutes of brisk walking. You can start with shorter durations and gradually increase as your fitness improves.

6. Cool Down: Slow down your pace in the last few minutes to allow your heart rate to gradually return to normal.

7. Stretch: Finish with some gentle stretching exercises for your leg muscles.

Cycling:

1. Adjust Bike: Set up your bike seat and handlebars to a comfortable position. Wear a helmet for safety.

2. Start Slow: Begin pedaling at a moderate pace to warm up for about 5-10 minutes.

3. Increase Intensity: Gradually increase your pedaling speed or resistance level to make it more challenging.

4. Maintain Form: Keep a relaxed grip on the handlebars, and maintain a neutral spine while cycling.

5. Vary Terrain: If cycling outdoors, vary the terrain by including flat roads, hills, or intervals of increased speed to add variety and intensity.

6. Duration: Aim for at least 20-30 minutes of continuous cycling. Increase duration as your fitness improves.

7. Cool Down: Slow down your pedaling and ride at an easy pace for a few minutes before stopping.

8. Stretch: Perform stretching exercises for your legs and lower back after cycling to prevent stiffness.

Swimming:

1. Warm-up: Start with a few laps at an easy pace to warm up your muscles and get comfortable in the water.
2. Choose Stroke: Use different strokes such as freestyle, breaststroke, backstroke, or butterfly, alternating between them for variety.
3. Control Breathing: Focus on rhythmic breathing, coordinating it with your strokes. Exhale when your face is in the water and inhale when turning your head to breathe.
4. Maintain Form: Work on your swimming technique, ensuring proper arm movements, kicks, and body position in the water.
5. Vary Intensity: Increase the intensity by swimming faster, doing intervals, or incorporating different strokes.
6. Duration: Aim for 20-30 minutes of continuous swimming, gradually increasing as your endurance improves.
7. Cool Down: Swim at an easy pace for a few laps to cool down before exiting the pool.

8. Stretch: Perform gentle stretching exercises focusing on the shoulders, back, and legs after swimming.

Remember, before starting any exercise routine, consult with a healthcare professional or fitness expert, especially if you have any health concerns or conditions. Adjust the intensity and duration of exercises based on your fitness level and gradually progress to more challenging workouts to avoid injury.

2. Strength Training:

Definition: Strength training, also known as resistance or weight training, involves using resistance or weights to challenge and strengthen muscles. While not directly targeting the cardiovascular system like aerobic exercises, it offers notable benefits for heart fitness.

Contributions to Heart Fitness:

- Improved Muscle Mass: Building and maintaining muscle mass through strength training helps increase the body's overall metabolic rate, contributing to better weight management and indirectly supporting heart health.

- Enhanced Cardiovascular Efficiency: Strength training, when performed with shorter rest intervals between sets or in a circuit-style format, can elevate the heart rate and maintain it within a moderate range, offering cardiovascular benefits.

- Better Blood Sugar Control: Regular strength training helps regulate blood sugar levels, which is crucial for overall heart health and reducing the risk of heart-related complications in individuals with diabetes.

- Examples: Exercises involving resistance bands, free weights, machines, bodyweight exercises (e.g., squats, lunges, push-ups), and functional movements fall under strength training categories.

Step-by-step guide for common strength training exercises:

1. Squats:

- Starting Position:
  - Stand with your feet shoulder-width apart, toes pointing slightly outward.
  - Keep your back straight, chest up, and core engaged.

- Execution:
  - Lower your body by bending your knees and hips, as if sitting back into an imaginary chair.
  - Keep your weight on your heels, and lower yourself until your thighs are parallel to the ground.

- Ensure your knees stay aligned with your toes and don't extend past your toes.
- Push through your heels to return to the starting position.

2. Push-Ups:

- Starting Position:
  - Begin in a plank position, with your hands slightly wider than shoulder-width apart.
  - Keep your body in a straight line from head to heels, engaging your core and glutes.

- Execution:
  - Lower your body towards the floor by bending your elbows, keeping them close to your body.
  - Lower until your chest nearly touches the ground, then push back up to the starting position.
  - Maintain a controlled movement, ensuring your body stays in a straight line throughout the exercise.

3. Lunges:

- Starting Position:
  - Stand tall with your feet together.
  - Take a step forward with one leg, keeping your torso upright.

- Execution:
  - Lower your body until both knees are bent at a 90-degree angle, ensuring the front knee is directly above your ankle.
  - The back knee should hover just above the ground.
  - Push back to the starting position by driving through the heel of your front foot.

4. Plank:

- Starting Position:
  - Begin in a prone position on the floor, resting on your forearms and toes.
  - Keep your elbows directly under your shoulders and your body in a straight line.

- Execution:

- Engage your core muscles to keep your body in a straight line from head to heels.
- Hold this position, ensuring your back remains flat and avoiding sagging or arching.
- Aim to hold for a specific duration based on your fitness level before resting.

5. Bent-Over Rows:

- Starting Position:
  - Stand with your feet shoulder-width apart, knees slightly bent.
  - Hold a dumbbell in each hand, palms facing your body, and hinge forward at the hips, keeping your back straight.

- Execution:
  - Pull the dumbbells towards your torso by bending your elbows and squeezing your shoulder blades together.
  - Lower the dumbbells back down to the starting position in a controlled manner.

Always prioritize proper form and technique over the number of repetitions or weight lifted to prevent injury and maximize effectiveness. If you're new to strength training, consider consulting with a fitness professional to ensure correct form and appropriate weights for your fitness level.

Sample exercise routines tailored for different fitness levels and age groups:

Exercise Routine for Beginners:

Note: Perform each exercise for 10-15 repetitions (reps) or 30-60 seconds, aiming for 1-2 sets initially. Gradually increase repetitions and sets as you progress.

1. Warm-Up:
   - 5 minutes of brisk walking or jogging in place.

2. Exercises:
   - Bodyweight Squats: 2 sets of 10-15 reps.
   - Knee Push-Ups: 2 sets of 10-15 reps.
   - Stationary Lunges: 2 sets of 10-12 reps per leg.

- Plank: Hold for 30-45 seconds.
- Bent-Over Rows (with resistance band or light dumbbells): 2 sets of 12-15 reps.

3. Cool Down:
- 5-10 minutes of stretching exercises targeting major muscle groups.

Exercise Routine for Intermediate Level:

Note: Perform each exercise for 12-20 reps or 45-60 seconds, aiming for 2-3 sets.

1. Warm-Up:
- 5-10 minutes of moderate cardio (jogging, cycling, or jump rope).

2. Exercises:
- Squats with Dumbbells: 3 sets of 12-15 reps.
- Push-Ups: 3 sets of 12-15 reps.

- Forward Lunges (with or without dumbbells): 3 sets of 12 reps per leg.
- Plank Variations (side plank, forearm plank): Hold for 45-60 seconds.
- Bent-Over Rows (with dumbbells): 3 sets of 12-15 reps.

3. Cool Down:
- 10 minutes of stretching exercises focusing on muscle groups used during the routine.

Exercise Routine for Seniors (Low-Impact):

Note: Perform exercises slowly and with controlled movements. Use resistance bands or light weights if comfortable.

1. Warm-Up:
- 5-7 minutes of walking or marching in place.

2. Exercises:
- Seated Marches: 2 sets of 20 reps (lifting knees while seated).

- Seated Leg Extensions (with resistance band): 2 sets of 12-15 reps per leg.
- Seated Rows (with resistance band or light dumbbells): 2 sets of 12-15 reps.
- Wall Push-Ups (standing, using a wall for support): 2 sets of 12-15 reps.
- Modified Plank (leaning against a kitchen counter): Hold for 20-30 seconds.

3. Cool Down:
- Gentle stretches targeting major muscle groups, holding each stretch for 20-30 seconds.

Always consult with a healthcare professional or fitness trainer before starting any exercise routine, especially if you have existing health conditions or concerns. Adjust the routines based on individual abilities and comfort levels.

Incorporating Physical Activity into Daily Life for a Healthier Heart

Leading a sedentary lifestyle can have adverse effects on cardiovascular health. Incorporating movement and physical activity into daily routines is essential for promoting heart health. Here are practical tips to infuse more activity into your everyday life:

1. Take Active Breaks: Instead of extended periods of sitting, take short breaks every hour. Stand up, stretch, or take a brief walk around your home or office to break up sedentary behavior.

2. Use Stairs: Opt for stairs instead of elevators whenever possible. Climbing stairs provides an excellent cardiovascular workout and engages various muscle groups.

3. Walk Whenever Feasible: Park farther away from your destination or get off public transport

a stop earlier to incorporate more walking into your daily routine.

4. Active Commuting: Consider cycling or walking to work, if feasible. This not only increases physical activity but also reduces reliance on motorized transport.

5. Lunchtime Walks: Use your lunch break to take a brisk walk. Invite colleagues to join for added motivation and social interaction.

6. Household Chores: Engage in household chores that involve movement, such as vacuuming, gardening, or washing the car. These activities contribute to burning calories and keeping active.

7. Standing Desk or Active Sitting: Consider using a standing desk or an adjustable desk that allows both sitting and standing. Incorporate active sitting by using an exercise ball instead of a chair to engage core muscles.

8. Take Active Leisure Time: Instead of passive activities like watching TV or browsing the internet, opt for activities that involve movement, such as dancing, playing outdoor games, or going for a family hike.

9. Set Activity Goals: Set achievable physical activity goals for each day. Start small and gradually increase duration and intensity as your fitness improves.

10. Join Group Activities: Participate in community-based activities or group fitness classes. It not only keeps you active but also provides social support and motivation.

11. Use Technology Smartly: Utilize fitness apps or wearable devices that track your steps, set reminders to move, or provide exercise routines to keep you motivated.

Incorporating physical activity into daily routines is an effective way to increase overall movement, improve heart health, and reduce the risks associated with a sedentary lifestyle. Making small, consistent changes can lead to significant improvements in cardiovascular fitness and overall well-being.

Chapter 4: Quitting Bad

Habits

Step-by-step guide to help you quit smoking:

Step 1: Set a Quit Date

- Choose a specific date within the next few weeks to quit smoking. This date serves as a goal and gives you time to mentally prepare.

Step 2: Prepare for Quit Day

- Discard all cigarettes, lighters, and ashtrays from your home, car, and workplace.

- Identify triggers that prompt you to smoke (stress, social situations, etc.) and plan alternatives to cope with these triggers.
- Inform friends, family, and coworkers about your decision to quit and request their support.

Step 3: Seek Support

- Consider joining a smoking cessation program, support group, or seeking guidance from a healthcare professional. Behavioral counseling can provide strategies to cope with cravings and withdrawal symptoms.

Step 4: Use Nicotine Replacement Therapy (NRT) or Medications

- Explore nicotine replacement therapies like patches, gum, lozenges, nasal sprays, or prescribed medications (varenicline, bupropion) to manage cravings and withdrawal symptoms. Follow recommended usage guidelines.

Step 5: Develop Coping Strategies

- Find healthy alternatives to smoking, such as chewing gum, drinking water, going for walks, or practicing relaxation techniques (deep breathing, meditation) to handle cravings and stress.

Step 6: Stay Active and Healthy

- Engage in regular physical activity to reduce stress and boost mood.
- Eat a balanced diet and drink plenty of water to maintain overall health and distract from cravings.

Step 7: Avoid Triggers and Temptations

- Stay away from situations, places, or people that may trigger the urge to smoke, especially during the initial quitting phase.
- Consider avoiding alcohol and other substances that can weaken your resolve to quit.

Step 8: Stay Positive and Persistent

- Understand that quitting smoking is a process that may involve setbacks. Don't get discouraged by slip-ups; instead, use them as learning opportunities.
- Stay positive and remind yourself of the benefits of quitting, such as improved health, saving money, and a smoke-free lifestyle.

Step 9: Reward Yourself

- Celebrate milestones and achievements in your journey to quit smoking. Treat yourself to rewards such as a movie, a book, or a relaxing activity for staying smoke-free.

Step 10: Stay Committed

- Stay committed to your decision to quit smoking, even if it's challenging. Remind yourself of your motivations and reasons for quitting.

Remember, everyone's quitting journey is unique. If you face difficulties or need additional support, don't hesitate to seek help from healthcare professionals, support groups, or counselors. With determination and support, quitting smoking is achievable, leading to improved health and well-being.

Step-by-Step Guide for Alcohol Cessation

1. Recognize the Need for Change:
   - Acknowledge the negative impact of alcohol on your life, health, relationships, or daily functioning. Understand why reducing or quitting alcohol is essential for your well-being.

2. Set Realistic Goals:
   - Define clear and achievable goals regarding alcohol reduction or cessation. Start with small, achievable steps, such as reducing the number of drinks per day or per week.

3. Create a Plan:
   - Develop a structured plan outlining your approach to cessation. Consider setting a quit date, deciding on strategies to cope with cravings, and identifying triggers that lead to drinking.

4. Seek Support:
   - Reach out to family, friends, or support groups for encouragement and accountability. Inform them about your decision and ask for their understanding and support during this transition.

5. Find Alternative Coping Strategies:
   - Identify healthy alternatives to manage stress or cope with situations that typically lead to drinking. Engage in activities like exercise, meditation, hobbies, or relaxation techniques.

6. Remove Temptations:
   - Rid your environment of alcohol. Discard any remaining alcohol from your home, avoid places or events that encourage drinking, and surround yourself with supportive influences.

7. Stay Hydrated and Eat Healthily:
   - Ensure you drink plenty of water and maintain a balanced diet. Proper hydration and nutrition can help alleviate withdrawal symptoms and maintain overall health.

8. Educate Yourself:
   - Learn about the effects of alcohol, withdrawal symptoms, and potential challenges you may face during the cessation process. Understanding what to expect can better prepare you for the journey.

9. Consider Professional Help:
   - Seek guidance from healthcare professionals, counselors, or addiction specialists. They can provide personalized support, counseling, or medical interventions, if necessary.

10. Monitor Progress and Celebrate Milestones:
    - Track your progress regularly. Celebrate achievements, whether big or small, and use them as motivation to continue on your path to alcohol cessation.

Step-by-step guide to gradually reduce sugar intake:

Step 1: Assess Current Sugar Intake

- Start by examining your current diet to understand how much sugar you consume daily. This includes not only obvious sources like sweets and sugary drinks but also hidden sugars in processed foods, sauces, dressings, and beverages.

Step 2: Identify High-Sugar Foods

- Make a list of foods high in added sugars. Common culprits include sugary beverages (sodas, energy drinks), candies, pastries, sugary cereals, desserts, and processed snacks.

Step 3: Educate Yourself on Hidden Sugars

- Learn to read food labels to identify hidden sugars. Ingredients like high-fructose corn syrup, maltose, dextrose, sucrose, and fruit juice concentrate indicate added sugars. Be aware that even seemingly healthy foods like flavored yogurt or granola bars can contain significant amounts of added sugars.

Step 4: Set Realistic Goals

- Establish achievable goals for reducing sugar intake. Aim to gradually cut down on added sugars rather than eliminating them all at once. Small, sustainable changes are more likely to lead to long-term success.

Step 5: Substitute with Natural Sweeteners

- Use natural sweeteners like stevia, monk fruit, or small amounts of honey or maple syrup as alternatives to refined sugars. However, moderation is key even with natural sweeteners.

Step 6: Choose Whole Foods

- Focus on whole foods like fruits, vegetables, whole grains, and lean proteins. These foods contain natural sugars and offer essential nutrients without the added sugars found in processed foods.

Step 7: Opt for Unsweetened Alternatives

- Choose unsweetened versions of beverages like tea, coffee, and almond milk. This reduces sugar intake without compromising flavor.

Step 8: Limit Processed Foods

- Minimize consumption of processed foods like canned soups, sauces, and pre-packaged meals, as they often contain hidden sugars. Cook meals at home using fresh ingredients whenever possible.

Step 9: Gradually Reduce Sugar in Recipes

- When cooking or baking, gradually reduce the amount of sugar in recipes. Experiment with using less sugar or substituting it with spices like cinnamon or nutmeg for added flavor.

Step 10: Monitor Progress and Adjust

- Keep track of your sugar intake and monitor your progress. Celebrate small victories and adjust your goals as needed. Be patient with yourself as you make these changes.

Chapter 5: Lifestyle Modifications for Heart Wellness

Stress Management: Techniques for Reducing Stress and its Impact on Heart Health

Stress, if left unmanaged, can significantly impact heart health and contribute to the development or exacerbation of cardiovascular conditions. Understanding effective stress management techniques is vital for maintaining a healthy heart. Here are several strategies to help reduce stress and its impact on heart health:

1. Mindfulness Meditation:
   - Practice mindfulness meditation to focus on the present moment, reduce anxiety, and alleviate stress. Meditation techniques involving controlled breathing and relaxation exercises can have a calming effect on both the mind and body.

2. Deep Breathing Exercises:

- Find a Comfortable Position:
  - Sit or lie down in a comfortable and quiet place. Ensure your back is straight but relaxed, allowing for natural breathing.

- Relax Your Body:
  - Close your eyes if it helps you focus and relax. Loosen any tense muscles in your shoulders, neck, and jaw.

- Take a Deep Breath In:
    - Inhale slowly and deeply through your nose. Aim to expand your abdomen rather than just filling your chest. Feel your stomach rise as you breathe in.

- Hold Your Breath:
    - Once you've taken a full breath, hold it for a brief moment. Hold for a count of 4 or 5 seconds, or for a duration that feels comfortable for you.

- Exhale Slowly:
    - Exhale slowly and completely through your mouth. Gently push out all the air from your lungs. You can use your lips pursed slightly if it helps control the airflow.

- Repeat the Process:

- Repeat this deep breathing cycle several times, ensuring each breath is slow, deep, and controlled.
- As you practice, try to lengthen the duration of each inhale, hold, and exhale gradually.

- Focus on Relaxation:
  - While breathing deeply, focus your attention on the sensation of the breath entering and leaving your body.
  - Imagine tension leaving your body with each exhale, promoting a sense of calmness and relaxation.

- Set a Duration:
  - Start with a session of 5-10 minutes. As you become more comfortable with the exercise, you can extend the duration to 15-20 minutes or longer.

- Practice Regularly:

- Incorporate this deep breathing exercise into your daily routine, ideally practicing it at the same time each day. Consistency is key to experiencing the benefits.

- Monitor Your Breathing:
    - Pay attention to your breath pattern throughout the day. Whenever feeling stressed or anxious, use deep breathing as a quick relaxation technique.

3. Regular Physical Activity:
 - Engaging in regular exercise not only benefits cardiovascular health but also acts as a stress reliever. Physical activity stimulates the release of endorphins, the body's natural mood elevators, reducing stress levels.

4. Establishing Boundaries and Time Management:

- Prioritize tasks, set realistic goals, and learn to say no when necessary to manage stress levels. Effective time management reduces feelings of being overwhelmed and minimizes stress.

5. Healthy Sleep Patterns:
 - Ensure adequate sleep by maintaining a regular sleep schedule. Quality sleep promotes physical and emotional well-being, helping the body recover from daily stressors.

6. Social Support and Connection:
 - Seek social support from friends, family, or support groups. Building strong social connections provides emotional support, reduces feelings of isolation, and helps manage stress.

7. Relaxation Techniques:
 - Practice relaxation techniques such as progressive muscle relaxation, guided imagery, or yoga. These methods help relax muscles, calm the mind, and alleviate stress.

8. Time for Enjoyable Activities:

- Dedicate time for hobbies or activities that bring joy and relaxation. Engaging in enjoyable pursuits fosters a sense of fulfillment and reduces stress.

9. Limiting Stressors:
   - Identify and limit exposure to stressors where possible. Strategies may involve time management, communication skills, or minimizing exposure to stressful environments.

10. Seeking Professional Help:
    - Consider seeking guidance from mental health professionals or counselors if stress becomes overwhelming or impacts daily functioning.

Sleep and Heart Health:

Understanding the Importance of

Quality Sleep

Quality sleep is fundamental to overall health, including cardiovascular wellness. Understanding the significance of adequate and restful sleep is crucial in maintaining a healthy heart. Here's an exploration of the importance of quality sleep and its effects on cardiovascular wellness:

1. Sleep Duration and Heart Health:

   - Restorative Function: Quality sleep allows the body to repair and rejuvenate. It plays a pivotal role in supporting cardiovascular health by giving the heart and blood vessels time to rest and recover.

- Sleep Duration: Studies suggest that both insufficient sleep (less than 7 hours per night) and excessive sleep may impact heart health. Striking a balance with an optimal sleep duration is crucial for heart wellness.

2. Influence on Heart Disease Risk:

  - Hypertension Risk: Inadequate sleep has been associated with an increased risk of hypertension. Chronic sleep deprivation may lead to higher blood pressure, which is a significant risk factor for heart diseases.

  - Impact on Heart Rhythm: Irregular sleep patterns or poor sleep quality can disrupt the body's internal clock (circadian rhythm), potentially affecting heart rhythm and increasing the risk of cardiovascular events.

3. Sleep and Inflammation:

  - Inflammatory Response: Poor sleep patterns may contribute to increased inflammation in the body, which is linked to the development and progression of heart diseases.

4. Sleep Apnea and Heart Health:

   - Obstructive Sleep Apnea (OSA): This sleep disorder, characterized by pauses in breathing or shallow breathing during sleep, is associated with an increased risk of hypertension, stroke, and heart failure. Managing OSA is crucial for maintaining heart health.

5. Quality Sleep Tips for Heart Wellness:

   - Establishing a Sleep Routine: Maintain a consistent sleep schedule, aiming for 7-9 hours of uninterrupted sleep per night.

   - Creating a Restful Environment: Ensure a comfortable sleep environment—quiet, dark, and at a comfortable temperature—to promote restful sleep.

- Limiting Stimulants Before Bed: Avoid caffeine, heavy meals, and electronics close to bedtime, as they can interfere with sleep quality.

- Prioritizing Relaxation Techniques: Engage in relaxation practices, such as deep breathing or meditation, before bedtime to promote better sleep quality.

Conclusion:

Let's recap the key points from each chapter:

Understanding Cardiovascular Health:
- Explored the anatomy of the heart, the cardiovascular system, common heart conditions, and modifiable risk factors contributing to heart diseases.

Dietary Plans for Heart Health:
- Detailed the benefits of heart-healthy diets such as the Mediterranean and DASH diets, emphasizing whole foods, reducing sugar intake, and managing sodium levels.

Exercise Routines for Cardiovascular Fitness:

- Provided exercise routines tailored to different fitness levels and age groups, emphasizing the importance of regular physical activity in maintaining heart health.

Managing Risk Factors:
- Explored the impact of alcohol cessation and sugar reduction on heart health, highlighting the importance of lifestyle modifications in managing risk factors.

Lifestyle Modifications for Heart Wellness:
- Emphasized the significance of quality sleep in supporting cardiovascular health, discussing its role in reducing heart disease risk and promoting overall wellness.

Personalized Cardiovascular Wellness Plan

1. Dietary Modifications:
- Goal: Increase intake of heart-healthy foods and reduce processed and high-sugar foods.
  - Action Steps:
    - Consume more fruits, vegetables, whole grains, and lean proteins.
    - Limit intake of saturated fats and trans fats.
    - Incorporate the Mediterranean diet by including olive oil, nuts, seeds, and fish rich in omega-3 fatty acids.
    - Reduce added sugar intake by avoiding sugary beverages and processed snacks.

2. Physical Activity:
- Goal: Establish a regular exercise routine to improve cardiovascular fitness.
  - Action Steps:
    - Aim for at least 150 minutes of moderate-intensity aerobic exercise per week.

- Include activities like brisk walking, cycling, swimming, or dancing.
- Incorporate strength training exercises at least twice a week to strengthen muscles.

3. Stress Management:
- Goal: Implement strategies to reduce stress levels and promote relaxation.
  - Action Steps:
  - Practice deep breathing exercises or mindfulness meditation for 10 minutes daily.
  - Engage in hobbies or activities that provide relaxation and enjoyment.
  - Prioritize time management and establish boundaries to reduce stressors.

4. Quality Sleep Improvement:
- Goal: Optimize sleep quality and duration for better heart health.
  - Action Steps:
  - Maintain a consistent sleep schedule, aiming for 7-9 hours of sleep each night.

- Create a conducive sleep environment by keeping the room dark, quiet, and at a comfortable temperature.
- Establish a relaxing bedtime routine, such as reading or taking a warm bath before sleep.

5. Risk Factor Management:
- Goal: Manage modifiable risk factors contributing to heart diseases.
  - Action Steps:
    - Quit smoking or using tobacco products.
    - Limit alcohol intake or aim for complete cessation.
    - Monitor blood pressure and cholesterol levels regularly as per healthcare provider's recommendations.
    - Seek treatment or manage conditions like diabetes or obesity effectively.

6. Regular Health Check-ups:
- Goal: Schedule routine medical check-ups to monitor heart health.
  - Action Steps:

- Schedule annual physical examinations and screenings for heart-related conditions.

- Follow-up with healthcare providers for necessary evaluations and tests.

7. Accountability and Support:
- Goal: Seek support and maintain accountability for following the wellness plan.
  - Action Steps:
  - Share the wellness plan with a family member, friend, or healthcare professional for encouragement and support.
  - Consider joining support groups or wellness communities for motivation and shared experiences.

Printed in Great Britain
by Amazon